AF431684

HEALING

HYPOTHYROIDISM

AN ULTIMATE TREATMENT
AND CURE OF
HYPOTHYROIDISM

DR. ETHAN BARTON

Table of Contents

CHAPTER ONE

HYPOTHYROIDISM

What is hypothyroidism, exactly?

Hypothyroidism is a condition in which your metabolism slows down due to a lack of thyroid hormone in your bloodstream.

In hypothyroidism, thyroid hormone production and release are insufficient for the body's needs. This slows down your entire body's metabolism, making you feel sluggish. Hypothyroidism, also referred to as thyroid underactivity disease, is a fairly common condition.

Myxedema occurs when your thyroid levels are extremely low. There are a number of potentially life-threatening symptoms associated with myxedema, including the following:

• A sluggish heartbeat.

• Anemia.

Failure of the heart.

• Confusion.

• Coma.

This type of hypothyroidism is extremely dangerous and can lead to death.

As a rule, hypothyroidism is a condition that can be successfully treated. Controlling it is as simple as taking prescribed medications on a regular basis and making follow-up appointments with your doctor.

What is the function of my thyroid?

Located in the front of your neck just below the vocal cords, the thyroid gland is a small, butterfly-shaped organ that helps regulate your metabolism (larynx). The butterfly's body is centered on your neck, with its wings swaddling your windpipe like a cocoon (trachea). The thyroid's primary function is to regulate your metabolic rate. It is through metabolism that food is converted into the energy your body needs to run. In order to regulate your metabolism, the thyroid produces the hormones T4 and T3. It is the job of these hormones to tell the cells of the body how much energy they should use. They're in charge of regulating your core temperature and heart rate, respectively.

As long as your thyroid is functioning properly, new hormones are being produced and released on a regular basis. You can maintain a healthy metabolism and all of your body's systems by doing this The pituitary gland, which is located in the center of the skull below the brain, regulates the amount of thyroid hormones in the bloodstream. Pituitary gland TSH (thyroid stimulating hormone) regulates thyroid hormone levels when the pituitary gland senses a deficiency or excess of the hormone.

The entire body is affected if the thyroid hormone levels are too high or low (hyperthyroidism or hypothyroidism).

Hypothyroidism affects whom?

People of any age, gender, or ethnicity can develop hypothyroidism. Especially in women over 60, this is a common problem. After menopause, women are more likely than at any other time in their lives to develop hypothyroidism.

CHAPTER TWO

Is hypothyroidism or hyperthyroidism more serious?

Hypothyroidism occurs when the thyroid produces too little thyroid hormone.

Hyperthyroidism and hypothyroidism are two different conditions because of the amount of thyroid hormone produced. Hypothyroidism is characterized by a deficiency in thyroid hormone production. Hyperthyroidism, on the other hand, occurs when the thyroid produces too much thyroid hormone. Thyroid hormone levels are elevated in hyperthyroidism, causing an increase in metabolism. Your metabolism slows down if you have hypothyroidism.

Between the two states, many things are polar opposites. Hypothyroidism can make it difficult to get over a cold. Hyperthyroidism can make it difficult to deal with the heat. In terms of thyroid function, they represent opposite ends of the spectrum. I would recommend a central location for your body. Both of these conditions have treatments aimed at restoring thyroid function as closely as possible to the middle ground.

Symptoms and causes

Why does one become hypothyroid?

It is possible for hypothyroidism to be caused by a primary or secondary issue. Low thyroid hormone levels can be caused by a variety of factors, but one of the most common is an ailment that directly affects the thyroid gland. The pituitary gland, which sends TSH to the thyroid, is a secondary cause of hypothyroidism because it is unable to function properly.

Hypothyroidism is more commonly caused by underlying medical conditions. A condition associated with the immune system known as Hashimoto's disease accounts for the majority of cases. Hereditary thyroiditis, or Hashimoto's thyroiditis, is also known as chronic lymphocytic thyroiditis (passed down through a family). Because the immune system attacks and damages the thyroid in Hashimoto's disease, As a result, the thyroid is unable to produce or release adequate amounts of thyroid hormone.

Hypothyroidism can also be caused by the following primary causes:

Thyroiditis (inflammation of the thyroid).

treatment for an overactive thyroid (radiation and surgical removal of the thyroid).

If you don't have enough iodine in your body, your thyroid will not be able to produce hormones.

Diseases that run in families (a medical condition passed down through your family).

Viruses and postpartum thyroiditis are two possible causes of thyroiditis.

CHAPTER THREE

Pregnancy-induced hypothyroidism: what are the causes?

Hashimoto's disease is the most common diagnosis for pregnant women who experience hypothyroidism. The immune system attacks and damages the thyroid gland in this autoimmune disease. This causes the thyroid to be unable to produce and release adequate amounts of thyroid hormones, which has an effect on the whole body. They may feel exhausted, have a difficult time coping with the cold, or suffer from muscle cramps.

When your baby is in the womb, thyroid hormones are critical. Helps develop the brain and nervous system by way of these hormones. Pregnancy thyroid monitoring is critical for women who have hypothyroidism or are at risk for it. It's possible that the brain won't develop properly in your baby if he or she doesn't get enough thyroid hormone during development. Hypothyroidism during pregnancy can cause miscarriage or premature labor if it is not properly treated.

What impact does the pill I'm taking to regulate my thyroid have?

The estrogen and progesterone in birth control pills can alter your thyroid-binding proteins if you're taking them. With this, you'll rise in the ranks Hypothyroidism may necessitate a higher dosage of your medication while taking birth control pills. You will need to lower the dosage after you stop taking birth control pills.

Is it possible that hypothyroidism can lead to impotence?

Untreated hypothyroidism may be linked to erectile dysfunction in some cases. Hypothyroidism can cause low testosterone levels if your pituitary gland is malfunctioning. If the hormone imbalance is the root cause of the erectile dysfunction, treating hypothyroidism often helps.

Hypothyroidism signs and symptoms

Hypothyroidism's symptoms usually appear gradually, sometimes over the course of several months or even years. They can include, but are not limited to:

- Tiredness is setting in (fatigue).

Your hands will feel numb, and tingling will be a constant presence.

• Constipation.

• Weight gain.

Feeling achy all over your body (can include muscle weakness).

• Having cholesterol levels in the blood that are higher than normal.

• I'm depressed right now.

Inability to tolerate cold weather.

The skin and hair are dry and brittle.

• Feeling less sexy as a result.

• Having menstrual cycles that are both frequent and heavy.

Becoming more aware of the way you look (including drooping eyelids, as well as puffiness in the eyes and face).

Your voice becoming hoarser and lower.

Forgetting things more frequently (brain fog).

I'm worried that hypothyroidism will cause me to put on weight.

You may gain weight if your hypothyroidism is not treated. Weight loss should begin as soon as you begin treating the condition. However, if you want to lose weight, you'll need to keep an eye on your caloric intake and get some exercise. Make an appointment with your doctor to discuss a weight loss plan that's right for you.

Tests and Diagnosis

What are the symptoms of hypothyroidism?

Symptoms of hypothyroidism can be easily mistaken for those of other conditions, making diagnosis difficult. Consult your physician if you experience any of the signs and symptoms of hypothyroidism. The thyroid stimulating hormone (TSH) test is the primary method for diagnosing hypothyroidism. Hashimoto's disease, for example, may warrant a blood test from your doctor. When your doctor performs a physical exam during an appointment, they may be able to detect an enlarged thyroid.

CHAPTER FOUR

CARE AND MANAGEMENT

What is the treatment for hypothyroidism?

Hypothyroidism is usually treated by supplementing the hormone your body isn't producing. Typically, a medication is used to accomplish this. Levothyroxine is one of the most commonly prescribed medications. Taken orally, this medication boosts your body's production of thyroid hormone, ensuring that your levels are stable.

In most cases, hypothyroidism is a treatable condition. You will, however, be on medication for the rest of your life in order to keep your hormone levels in check. You can lead a normal and healthy life with proper management and follow-up appointments with your healthcare provider.

Hypothyroidism can lead to a variety of health problems.

It's possible that untreated hypothyroidism will worsen to the point where it's life-threatening. If you don't get help, you could develop more serious symptoms, such as:

• The emergence of mental health issues.

• I'm struggling to breathe.

Body temperature cannot be maintained. •

Concerns about one's heart health.

• Creating a goiter (enlargement of the thyroid gland).

Myxedema coma is a life-threatening medical condition that can occur. If hypothyroidism is not addressed, this can occur.

Is my hypothyroidism medication regimen going to be the same for the rest of my life?

As your body adjusts to the medication, your dosage may need to be adjusted as well. The dosage of your medication may need to be adjusted as your symptoms change over time. This can occur as a result of changes in body composition, such as weight gain or loss. To ensure that your medication is working properly, you will need to have your levels monitored throughout your life.

PREVENTION

Is it possible to prevent hypothyroidism?

There is no way to avoid developing hypothyroidism. Watching for signs of hypothyroidism is the best way to avoid developing a serious form of the condition or having its symptoms seriously impact your life. Health care providers can help diagnose hypothyroidism, so if you notice any of the symptoms, don't hesitate to get in touch! If you catch hypothyroidism early and begin treatment, it is manageable.

LIVING IN CONNECTION WITH

Please tell me if there are any foods that can help my hypothyroidism.

You don't have to worry about your iodine intake because most foods in Western diets contain it. Iodine is a mineral that aids in the production of hormones by your thyroid. There is some evidence to suggest that increasing your intake of iodine-rich foods, if you suffer from low thyroid hormone levels, may help. Increases in hormone levels can only be achieved through the use of a prescription medication, available only through your physician. Talk to your doctor before embarking on a new diet. Before embarking on a new diet, especially if you have a medical condition like hypothyroidism, it is critical to speak with your doctor.

Foods high in iodine include:.

• Eggs.

There are a wide variety of dairy products available.

• Fish, shellfish, and poultry.

Eating seaweed. •

• Salt that has been iodized.

Make a meal plan with the help of your doctor or a nutritionist (a doctor who specializes in food). Your food is the fuel that powers you through the day. Maintaining a healthy diet and taking your prescribed medication as prescribed can help you live a long and healthy life. As a precaution, people with a thyroid disorder should avoid taking in large amounts of iodine (self-contradictory).

The answer to this question is a resounding yes.

Hypothyroidism symptoms may not appear at all, or they may lessen with time if you have a mild case. Hypothyroidism symptoms may persist for weeks or months after starting treatment, but this is not always the case. Hypothyroidism is a long-term condition that requires regular medication for those with low levels of thyroid hormones. Hypothyroidism can be managed effectively and you can lead a normal life despite the condition.

THE END

www.ingramcontent.com/pod-product-compliance
Lightning Source LLC
Chambersburg PA
CBHW050622160726
48003CB00003B/1293